MODERN METHODS FOR MASTERING MASA

Discover Revolutionary Techniques, Tempting Recipes, and Thoughtful Reflections on the Timeless Staple.

MICHAEL JUNIOR

TABLE OF CONTENT

Introduction

"Modern Methods for Mastering Masa: Discover Revolutionary Techniques, Tempting Recipes, and Thoughtful Reflections on the Timeless Staple" is a thorough reference that unveils the mysteries of masa, a classic maize dough used in Latin American and Mexican cuisine.

Masa has a long and rich cultural past, and it serves as the foundation for a wide range of foods, from traditional tortillas and tamales to a wide range of modern inventions.

This book will teach you how to master masa using current techniques, inventive twists, and time-tested principles, allowing you to create great masa-based meals in your own kitchen.

From classic favorites to modern fusions, you'll find a wide selection of recipes that highlight the flexibility of masa.

Each recipe is meticulously tailored to highlight the flavor and texture of this time-honored favorite. These recipes will inspire you to release your creativity and satisfy your palate, whether you are an expert cook or a beginner wishing to extend your culinary talents.

Furthermore, this book is about more than just cooking; it's about the culture, history, and joy that masa gives to the world of food.

Throughout the book, there are thoughtful notes that inspire you to investigate the tales and origins of the recipes, as well as to understand the cultural significance of masa in the culinary environment.

Join us on this culinary trip as we discover the wonders of masa, experiment with new techniques, savor delectable meals, and appreciate the ageless staple's significant effect.

Masa Crepes with Berries and Cream

Ingredients:

For the Crepes:

- 1 cup masa harina
- 2 cups milk
- 2 large eggs
- Pinch of salt
- 2 tablespoons melted butter (for the batter)
- Additional butter or oil for cooking

For the Filling:

- Mixed berries (strawberries, blueberries, raspberries)
- Whipped cream
- Honey or maple syrup for drizzling (optional)

Method:

1. **Prepare the Crepe Batter:**
   - In a mixing bowl, combine the masa harina, milk, eggs, salt, and melted butter.

- Whisk the ingredients until you have a smooth, thin batter.

2. **Cook the Crepes:**

   - Heat a non-stick skillet or crepe pan over medium heat and add a small amount of butter or oil to coat the surface.

   - Pour a small amount of batter into the center of the pan, swirling it to spread thinly.

   - Cook for about 1-2 minutes per side until the edges are golden brown. Repeat until all the batter is used.

3. **Prepare the Filling:**

   - Wash and slice the berries as needed.

   - Whip the cream until soft peaks form.

4. **Assemble the Crepes:**

   - Lay a crepe flat on a plate.

   - Add a generous spoonful of whipped cream in the center of the crepe.

   - Scatter a handful of mixed berries over the whipped cream.

5. **Fold and Serve:**

  - Fold the crepe over the filling, creating a half-moon shape.

  - Repeat with the remaining crepes and filling.

  - Drizzle with honey or maple syrup if desired.

Benefits:

1. **Masa Harina:**

  - Rich in fiber, providing digestive benefits.

  - Contains essential nutrients like iron, zinc, and B vitamins.

2. **Berries:**

  - Packed with antioxidants that help fight inflammation and support overall health.

  - High in vitamins C and K, as well as fiber.

3. **Whipped Cream:**

  - Provides a source of calcium and vitamin D for bone health.

  - Adds a delightful, creamy texture to the crepes.

4. **Honey or Maple Syrup (optional):**

- Natural sweeteners with potential antioxidant and anti-inflammatory properties.

- Can add a touch of sweetness without refined sugars.

Cornbread Masa Stuffing

Ingredients:

For the Cornbread:

- 1 cup masa harina
- 1 cup cornmeal
- 1 cup all-purpose flour
- 1 tablespoon baking powder
- 1 teaspoon salt
- 1 cup buttermilk
- 2 large eggs
- 1/2 cup unsalted butter, melted
- 1/4 cup honey

For the Stuffing:

- 4 cups cubed cornbread (prepared in advance)
- 1 cup diced celery
- 1 cup diced onion
- 1 cup diced apple
- 1/2 cup chopped fresh parsley
- 1 teaspoon dried sage
- 1 teaspoon dried thyme

- 2 cups chicken or vegetable broth
- Salt and pepper to taste

Method:

1. **Prepare the Cornbread:**

   - Preheat the oven to 375°F (190°C).

   - In a large bowl, combine masa harina, cornmeal, flour, baking powder, and salt.

   - In another bowl, whisk together buttermilk, eggs, melted butter, and honey.

   - Pour the wet ingredients into the dry ingredients and stir until just combined.

   - Pour the batter into a greased baking dish and bake for 20-25 minutes or until a toothpick comes out clean.

   - Allow the cornbread to cool, then cut it into cubes.

2. **Prepare the Stuffing:**

   - In a large skillet, sauté the celery, onion, and apple until softened.

- Add the dried sage and thyme, stirring to combine.

- In a large mixing bowl, combine the cubed cornbread, sautéed vegetables, and chopped parsley.

- Season with salt and pepper to taste.

3. **Bake the Stuffing:**

- Preheat the oven to 350°F (175°C).

- Pour the chicken or vegetable broth over the cornbread mixture and gently toss until evenly moistened.

- Transfer the stuffing to a greased baking dish and bake for 30-35 minutes or until the top is golden and crisp.

Benefits:

1. **Masa Harina:**

- Contains fiber, aiding in digestion.

- Rich in essential nutrients like iron and B vitamins.

2. **Cornbread:**

- A good source of carbohydrates for energy.

- Provides some protein and dietary fiber.

3. **Celery:**

    - Low in calories and high in fiber.

    - Contains vitamins A and K, as well as antioxidants.

4. **Onion:**

    - Adds flavor and contains antioxidants.

    - May have anti-inflammatory and immune-boosting properties.

5. **Apple:**

    - Adds natural sweetness and provides dietary fiber.

    - Rich in vitamin C and various antioxidants.

6. **Parsley:**

    - Contains vitamins A and C.

    - Acts as a fresh and flavorful herb in the stuffing.

7. **Sage and Thyme:**

    - Herbs with potential antioxidant and anti-inflammatory properties.

- Add aromatic flavor to the stuffing.

8. **Chicken or Vegetable Broth:**

- Adds moisture and flavor to the stuffing.

- May provide additional nutrients depending on the broth used.

Enjoy this Cornbread Masa Stuffing as a delicious side dish during holiday gatherings or as a comforting addition to any meal!

Masa Dumplings in Broth

Ingredients:

For the Dumplings:

- 1 cup masa harina
- 1/2 cup all-purpose flour
- 1 teaspoon baking powder
- 1/2 teaspoon salt
- 1/2 cup ground pork or plant-based alternative
- 1 tablespoon finely chopped fresh ginger
- 1/4 cup chopped green onions
- 1 large egg
- 1/4 cup water (adjust as needed)

For the Broth:

- 4 cups chicken or vegetable broth
- 1 cup sliced carrots
- 1 cup sliced bok choy or Napa cabbage
- 1 tablespoon soy sauce
- 1 teaspoon sesame oil
- Salt and pepper to taste

Method:

1. **Prepare the Dumplings:**

   - In a large mixing bowl, combine masa harina, all-purpose flour, baking powder, and salt.

   - Add ground pork (or plant-based alternative), chopped ginger, green onions, egg, and water. Mix until a sticky dough forms.

   - With wet hands, shape the dough into small, bite-sized dumplings.

2. **Cook the Dumplings:**

   - Bring a pot of water to a gentle boil.

   - Drop the dumplings into the boiling water and cook until they float to the surface (about 5 minutes).

   - Remove the dumplings with a slotted spoon and set aside.

3. **Prepare the Broth:**

   - In a separate pot, bring chicken or vegetable broth to a simmer.

   - Add sliced carrots and cook until slightly tender.

- Stir in sliced bok choy or Napa cabbage and continue to simmer until vegetables are cooked but still vibrant.

4. **Combine Dumplings and Broth:**

   - Carefully add the cooked dumplings to the simmering broth.

   - Season with soy sauce, sesame oil, salt, and pepper. Adjust seasoning to taste.

5. **Serve:**

   - Ladle the dumplings and broth into serving bowls.

   - Garnish with additional chopped green onions, if desired.

Benefits:

1. **Masa Harina:**

   - Contains dietary fiber and essential nutrients like iron and B vitamins.

2. **Ground Pork or Plant-Based Alternative:**

   - Provides a source of protein for muscle maintenance and repair.

3. **Ginger:**

  - Adds flavor and may have anti-inflammatory and digestive benefits.

4. **Green Onions:**

  - Low in calories and rich in vitamins K and C.

  - Adds a fresh, aromatic element to the dumplings.

5. **Carrots:**

  - Rich in beta-carotene, a precursor to vitamin A.

  - Provides antioxidants and supports eye health.

6. **Bok Choy or Napa Cabbage:**

  - Low in calories and high in vitamins A and C.

  - Adds a crisp texture to the broth.

7. **Chicken or Vegetable Broth:**

  - Hydrating and can provide additional nutrients depending on the type used.

  - Creates a flavorful base for the dumplings.

8. **Soy Sauce:**

   - Adds savory umami flavor to the broth.

9. **Sesame Oil:**

   - Enhances the overall flavor and adds a nutty aroma.

This Masa Dumplings in Broth recipe combines comforting dumplings with a flavorful broth for a satisfying and nutritious dish. Enjoy it as a warming meal during colder seasons.

Masa-Crusted Chicken Pot Pie

Ingredients:

For the Masa Crust:

- 1 cup masa harina
- 1 cup all-purpose flour
- 1/2 teaspoon salt
- 1/2 cup unsalted butter, cold and cubed
- 1/4 cup cold water (adjust as needed)

For the Filling:

- 2 cups cooked chicken, shredded
- 1 cup diced carrots
- 1 cup frozen peas
- 1 cup diced potatoes
- 1/2 cup diced celery
- 1/4 cup unsalted butter
- 1/3 cup all-purpose flour
- 2 cups chicken broth
- 1 cup milk
- Salt and pepper to taste
- 1 teaspoon dried thyme

- 1 teaspoon dried rosemary

Method:

1. **Prepare the Masa Crust:**

   - In a food processor, combine masa harina, all-purpose flour, and salt.

   - Add cold, cubed butter and pulse until the mixture resembles coarse crumbs.

   - Gradually add cold water, pulsing until the dough comes together.

   - Form the dough into a disc, wrap in plastic wrap, and refrigerate for at least 30 minutes.

2. **Prepare the Filling:**

   - In a large skillet, melt butter over medium heat.

   - Add diced carrots, peas, potatoes, and celery. Cook until vegetables are slightly tender.

   - Stir in the cooked shredded chicken.

   - Sprinkle flour over the mixture and stir to coat the ingredients.

3. **Create the Sauce:**

   - Gradually add chicken broth and milk, stirring continuously to avoid lumps.

   - Bring the mixture to a simmer until the sauce thickens.

   - Season with salt, pepper, dried thyme, and dried rosemary. Adjust seasoning to taste.

4. **Assemble the Pot Pie:**

   - Preheat the oven to 400°F (200°C).

   - Roll out the chilled masa dough on a floured surface to fit your pie dish.

   - Transfer the rolled-out dough to the pie dish, leaving excess hanging over the edges.

   - Pour the chicken and vegetable filling into the crust.

5. **Bake:**

   - Fold the excess masa dough over the top of the filling, creating a rustic, free-form crust.

   - Bake in the preheated oven for 25-30 minutes or until the crust is golden brown.

Benefits:

1. **Masa Harina:**

   - Adds a nutty flavor and contains dietary fiber, iron, and B vitamins.

2. **Chicken:**

   - A good source of lean protein for muscle health and repair.

   - Provides essential amino acids and various vitamins and minerals.

3. **Carrots, Peas, Potatoes, Celery:**

   - Rich in vitamins, minerals, and dietary fiber.

   - Contribute to the overall nutritional content of the pot pie.

4. **Butter and Flour:**

   - Provide richness and help create a creamy, savory filling.

   - Add flavor and contribute to the texture of the sauce.

5. **Chicken Broth:**

   - Adds depth of flavor and provides hydration.

- May contain nutrients extracted from the chicken during the cooking process.

6. **Milk:**

   - Adds creaminess and contributes to the overall texture of the filling.

   - Provides calcium and vitamin D.

7. **Thyme and Rosemary:**

   - Herbs with potential antioxidant and anti-inflammatory properties.

   - Enhance the flavor profile of the pot pie.

This Masa-Crusted Chicken Pot Pie is a hearty and comforting dish, perfect for a family dinner or a cozy gathering. Enjoy the warm, savory flavors and the unique twist of the masa crust.

Pumpkin Spice Tamales

Ingredients:

For the Masa Dough:

- 2 cups masa harina
- 1 cup pumpkin puree
- 1/2 cup unsalted butter, softened
- 1/2 cup brown sugar
- 1 teaspoon ground cinnamon
- 1/2 teaspoon ground ginger
- 1/4 teaspoon ground nutmeg
- 1/4 teaspoon ground cloves
- 1 teaspoon baking powder
- 1/2 teaspoon salt
- 1 1/2 cups vegetable broth

For the Filling:

- 1 cup sweetened condensed milk
- 1 cup finely chopped pecans or walnuts
- 1/2 cup raisins

For the Corn Husks:

- Dried corn husks, soaked in warm water until pliable

Method:

1. **Prepare the Masa Dough:**

   - In a large mixing bowl, combine masa harina, pumpkin puree, softened butter, brown sugar, ground cinnamon, ground ginger, ground nutmeg, ground cloves, baking powder, and salt.

   - Gradually add vegetable broth while stirring until a smooth, spreadable consistency is achieved.

2. **Prepare the Corn Husks:**

   - Soak dried corn husks in warm water for at least 30 minutes until they become pliable.

3. **Assemble the Tamales:**

   - Take a soaked corn husk and spread a thin layer of the pumpkin spice masa dough onto the center, leaving space around the edges.

   - Spoon a small amount of sweetened condensed milk onto the masa, then sprinkle chopped nuts and raisins over the top.

- Fold the sides of the husk toward the center and fold up the bottom. Tie with kitchen twine if needed.

4. **Steam the Tamales:**

   - Arrange the tamales vertically in a steamer basket, open side up.

   - Steam over boiling water for 1 to 1.5 hours or until the masa is set and easily pulls away from the husk.

5. **Serve:**

   - Allow the tamales to cool slightly before serving.

   - Optionally, drizzle with additional sweetened condensed milk and sprinkle with nuts before serving.

Benefits:

1. **Masa Harina:**

   - Contains dietary fiber, iron, and B vitamins.

2. **Pumpkin Puree:**

   - Rich in beta-carotene, which converts to vitamin A in the body.

   - Provides antioxidants and supports immune health.

3. **Butter and Brown Sugar:**

- Add richness and sweetness to the masa dough.

- Contribute to the overall flavor and texture of the tamales.

4. **Ground Cinnamon, Ginger, Nutmeg, Cloves:**

- Spices with potential anti-inflammatory and antioxidant properties.

- Add warm, comforting flavors to the tamales.

5. **Sweetened Condensed Milk:**

- Adds sweetness and creaminess to the filling.

- Provides a source of calcium and sugars for energy.

6. **Pecans or Walnuts:**

- Good sources of healthy fats, protein, and essential nutrients.

- Add a crunchy texture and nutty flavor to the tamales.

7. **Raisins:**

- Provide natural sweetness and contribute to the overall texture.

- Contain fiber, vitamins, and minerals.

These Pumpkin Spice Tamales offer a delightful twist on traditional tamales, combining the warmth of pumpkin spice with the rich flavors of sweetened condensed milk and nuts. Enjoy these as a festive treat during the fall and winter seasons.

Masa-Crusted Eggplant Parmesan

Ingredients:

For the Masa Crust:

- 1 cup masa harina
- 1 cup Italian-style breadcrumbs
- 1 teaspoon dried oregano
- 1 teaspoon dried basil
- 1/2 teaspoon garlic powder
- Salt and pepper to taste
- 2 large eggs, beaten
- 1 large eggplant, sliced into rounds

For the Eggplant Parmesan:

- 2 cups marinara sauce
- 2 cups shredded mozzarella cheese
- 1/2 cup grated Parmesan cheese
- Fresh basil leaves for garnish

Method:

1. **Prepare the Masa Crust:**
   - In a shallow bowl, combine masa harina, Italian-style breadcrumbs,

dried oregano, dried basil, garlic powder, salt, and pepper.

- Dip each eggplant round into the beaten eggs, then coat it evenly with the masa mixture, pressing gently to adhere.

2. **Bake the Masa-Crusted Eggplant:**

- Preheat the oven to 400°F (200°C).

- Place the coated eggplant rounds on a baking sheet lined with parchment paper.

- Bake for 15-20 minutes or until the crust is golden and the eggplant is tender.

3. **Assemble the Eggplant Parmesan:**

- In a baking dish, spread a thin layer of marinara sauce.

- Arrange the baked masa-crusted eggplant rounds over the sauce.

- Sprinkle shredded mozzarella and grated Parmesan over each eggplant round.

- Repeat the layers until all ingredients are used, finishing with a generous layer of cheese on top.

4. **Bake until Cheese is Melted:**

- Bake in the preheated oven for an additional 20-25 minutes or until the cheese is melted and bubbly.

5. **Serve:**

- Allow the Masa-Crusted Eggplant Parmesan to cool for a few minutes before slicing.

- Garnish with fresh basil leaves before serving.

Benefits:

1. **Masa Harina:**

- Adds a unique, nutty flavor and provides dietary fiber, iron, and B vitamins.

2. **Eggplant:**

- Low in calories and rich in fiber.

- Contains antioxidants, vitamins, and minerals.

3. **Italian-Style Breadcrumbs:**

- Adds a crispy texture to the eggplant.

- Provides carbohydrates for energy.

4. **Dried Oregano and Basil:**

- Herbs with potential antioxidant and anti-inflammatory properties.

- Enhance the overall flavor of the crust.

5. **Garlic Powder:**

- Adds savory flavor to the masa crust.

- May have antimicrobial and heart-healthy properties.

6. **Eggs:**

- Provide protein and contribute to the binding of the masa crust.

7. **Marinara Sauce:**

- Contains tomatoes rich in vitamins, antioxidants, and lycopene.

- Adds flavor and moisture to the dish.

8. **Mozzarella and Parmesan Cheese:**

- Good sources of calcium and protein.

- Contribute to the rich and cheesy texture of the Eggplant Parmesan.

9. **Fresh Basil:**

- Adds a burst of fresh flavor and contains vitamins A and K.

This Masa-Crusted Eggplant Parmesan is a creative twist on a classic dish, offering a gluten-free alternative with the added benefits of masa harina. Enjoy this hearty and flavorful meal as a satisfying dinner option.

Huitlacoche Quesadillas

Ingredients:

For the Quesadilla Filling:

- 2 cups huitlacoche (cuitlacoche) - Mexican corn truffle
- 1 tablespoon vegetable oil
- 1/2 cup diced onion
- 2 cloves garlic, minced
- Salt and pepper to taste

For the Quesadilla Assembly:

- Corn tortillas
- Shredded Oaxaca cheese or Mexican cheese blend
- Chopped fresh cilantro for garnish
- Lime wedges for serving

Method:

1. **Prepare the Huitlacoche Filling:**
   - In a skillet, heat vegetable oil over medium heat.
   - Add diced onion and sauté until translucent.

- Add minced garlic and huitlacoche to the skillet, stirring occasionally.

- Cook until the huitlacoche is tender and any excess liquid has evaporated.

- Season with salt and pepper to taste.

2. **Assemble the Quesadillas:**

   - Heat a separate skillet or griddle over medium heat.

   - Place a corn tortilla on the hot surface and sprinkle a generous amount of shredded Oaxaca cheese or Mexican cheese blend on one half of the tortilla.

   - Spoon some of the cooked huitlacoche mixture over the cheese.

   - Fold the tortilla in half, creating a half-moon shape, and press down gently with a spatula.

   - Cook until the cheese is melted and the tortilla is golden brown on both sides.

3. **Serve:**

- Repeat the process for the remaining tortillas and huitlacoche filling.

- Garnish the huitlacoche quesadillas with chopped fresh cilantro.

- Serve hot with lime wedges on the side.

Benefits:

1. **Huitlacoche (Cuitlacoche):**

- Rich in protein, vitamins, and minerals.

- Contains lysine, an amino acid often deficient in corn, and may have antioxidant properties.

2. **Onion and Garlic:**

- Provide flavor and depth to the filling.

- Contain antioxidants and may have various health benefits, including anti-inflammatory properties.

3. **Corn Tortillas:**

- Gluten-free and a good source of carbohydrates.

- Contain fiber and essential nutrients.

4. **Oaxaca Cheese or Mexican Cheese Blend:**

   - Good sources of calcium and protein.

   - Contribute to the creamy texture and cheesy flavor of the quesadillas.

5. **Cilantro:**

   - Adds a fresh and herbaceous flavor.

   - Contains antioxidants and may have antibacterial properties.

6. **Lime:**

   - Provides acidity and enhances the overall taste.

   - Rich in vitamin C and antioxidants.

Huitlacoche quesadillas offer a unique and earthy flavor that pairs well with the creamy cheese and fresh cilantro. Enjoy these quesadillas as a delicious and culturally rich dish in your Mexican cuisine repertoire.

Masa Waffles with Chicken and Mole

Ingredients:

For the Masa Waffles:

- 2 cups masa harina
- 1 tablespoon sugar
- 1 tablespoon baking powder
- 1/2 teaspoon salt
- 2 cups buttermilk
- 2 large eggs
- 1/4 cup unsalted butter, melted
- Cooking spray or additional butter for waffle iron

For the Chicken and Mole:

- 2 cups cooked and shredded chicken
- 1 cup mole sauce (store-bought or homemade)
- Chopped fresh cilantro for garnish
- Sesame seeds for garnish
- Lime wedges for serving

Method:

1. **Prepare the Masa Waffles:**

   - Preheat your waffle iron according to the manufacturer's instructions.

   - In a large bowl, whisk together masa harina, sugar, baking powder, and salt.

   - In a separate bowl, whisk together buttermilk, eggs, and melted butter.

   - Pour the wet ingredients into the dry ingredients and stir until just combined.

   - Lightly coat the waffle iron with cooking spray or butter.

   - Ladle the batter onto the hot waffle iron and cook until golden and crisp.

2. **Prepare the Chicken and Mole:**

   - In a saucepan, heat the shredded chicken with mole sauce over medium heat until warmed through.

   - Stir well to ensure the chicken is evenly coated with the mole sauce.

3. **Serve:**

- Place a Masa Waffle on a serving plate.
- Top with a generous portion of the chicken and mole mixture.
- Garnish with chopped cilantro and sesame seeds.
- Serve with lime wedges on the side.

Benefits:

1. **Masa Harina:**

- Adds a unique, nutty flavor and provides dietary fiber, iron, and B vitamins.

2. **Buttermilk:**

- Adds a tangy flavor to the waffles.
- Contains calcium, vitamin D, and probiotics.

3. **Eggs:**

- Provide protein and contribute to the structure of the waffles.

4. **Chicken:**

- A lean source of protein, supporting muscle health and repair.

- Provides essential amino acids and various vitamins and minerals.

5. **Mole Sauce:**

   - Contains a blend of rich flavors, including chocolate, chili peppers, and spices.

   - May contain antioxidants and provide unique depth to the dish.

6. **Cilantro:**

   - Adds a fresh and herbaceous flavor.

   - Contains antioxidants and may have antibacterial properties.

7. **Sesame Seeds:**

   - Provide a nutty flavor and a crunchy texture.

   - Rich in healthy fats, protein, and various nutrients.

8. **Lime:**

   - Adds acidity and brightness to the dish.

   - Rich in vitamin C and enhances flavor.

Masa-Crusted Avocado Fries

Ingredients:

For the Masa Coating:

- 1 cup masa harina
- 1 teaspoon chili powder
- 1/2 teaspoon garlic powder
- 1/2 teaspoon onion powder
- 1/2 teaspoon cumin
- 1/2 teaspoon salt
- 1/4 teaspoon black pepper
- 1 cup cold water
- 2 large avocados, peeled, pitted, and sliced into wedges

For Breading and Frying:

- 1 cup all-purpose flour
- 2 large eggs, beaten
- Cooking oil for frying (vegetable or avocado oil)

For Dipping Sauce:

- 1/2 cup plain Greek yogurt
- 1 tablespoon lime juice

- 1 tablespoon chopped fresh cilantro

- Salt and pepper to taste

Method:

1. **Prepare the Masa Coating:**

   - In a bowl, whisk together masa harina, chili powder, garlic powder, onion powder, cumin, salt, and black pepper.

   - Gradually add cold water, stirring until you have a smooth batter.

2. **Coat Avocado Slices:**

   - Dredge each avocado wedge in all-purpose flour, then dip into the beaten eggs.

   - Coat the avocado wedge in the masa batter, ensuring an even and thick coating.

3. **Fry the Avocado Fries:**

   - In a large skillet, heat cooking oil over medium heat.

   - Carefully place the coated avocado wedges in the hot oil and fry until golden brown on all sides.

- Transfer to a paper towel-lined plate to drain excess oil.

4. **Prepare the Dipping Sauce:**

   - In a small bowl, mix together Greek yogurt, lime juice, chopped cilantro, salt, and pepper.

   - Adjust the seasoning according to taste.

5. **Serve:**

   - Arrange the Masa-Crusted Avocado Fries on a serving platter.

   - Serve with the creamy lime cilantro dipping sauce on the side.

Benefits:

1. **Masa Harina:**

   - Adds a unique flavor and provides dietary fiber, iron, and B vitamins.

2. **Avocado:**

   - Packed with healthy monounsaturated fats.

   - Rich in vitamins K, C, E, and B-complex vitamins.

3. **Chili Powder, Garlic Powder, Onion Powder, Cumin:**

   - Spices with potential anti-inflammatory and antioxidant properties.

   - Add flavor and depth to the masa coating.

4. **Flour and Eggs:**

   - Create a coating that helps the masa adhere to the avocado slices.

   - Contribute to the overall texture and crispiness.

5. **Cooking Oil:**

   - Provides the necessary medium for frying.

   - May contain healthy unsaturated fats.

6. **Greek Yogurt:**

   - A rich source of protein and probiotics.

   - Creates a creamy base for the dipping sauce.

7. **Lime Juice:**

   - Adds acidity and brightness to the dipping sauce.

   - Rich in vitamin C and enhances flavor.

8. **Cilantro:**

   - Adds a fresh and herbaceous flavor to the dipping sauce.

   - Contains antioxidants and may have antibacterial properties.

Masa-Crusted Avocado Fries with Creamy Lime Cilantro Dipping Sauce offer a delightful combination of creamy avocado with a crispy, flavorful coating. Enjoy these fries as a tasty and unique appetizer or snack.

Spicy Masa Empanadas

Ingredients:

For the Masa Dough:

- 2 cups masa harina
- 1 teaspoon baking powder
- 1/2 teaspoon salt
- 1/2 cup unsalted butter, softened
- 1 cup warm chicken or vegetable broth

For the Spicy Filling:

- 1 tablespoon vegetable oil
- 1 cup diced onion
- 1 cup diced bell peppers (mixed colors)
- 1 cup cooked and shredded chicken or black beans for a vegetarian option
- 1 teaspoon ground cumin
- 1 teaspoon chili powder
- 1/2 teaspoon smoked paprika
- Salt and pepper to taste
- 1/4 cup chopped fresh cilantro
- 1/2 cup shredded Monterey Jack or pepper jack cheese

For Egg Wash:

- 1 egg, beaten

Method:

1. **Prepare the Masa Dough:**

   - In a large bowl, combine masa harina, baking powder, and salt.

   - Add softened butter and mix until crumbly.

   - Gradually add warm chicken or vegetable broth, kneading until you have a soft, pliable dough.

   - Cover the dough with a damp cloth and let it rest while preparing the filling.

2. **Prepare the Spicy Filling:**

   - In a skillet, heat vegetable oil over medium heat.

   - Add diced onion and bell peppers, sautéing until softened.

   - Add shredded chicken (or black beans), ground cumin, chili powder, smoked paprika, salt, and pepper. Cook until well combined.

- Stir in chopped cilantro and shredded cheese, allowing it to melt into the filling.

- Remove from heat and let the filling cool slightly.

3. **Assemble the Empanadas:**

   - Preheat the oven to 375°F (190°C).

   - Divide the masa dough into golf ball-sized portions.

   - Roll each portion into a ball and flatten it into a disk on a lightly floured surface.

   - Place a spoonful of the spicy filling in the center of each masa disk.

   - Fold the dough over the filling, creating a half-moon shape, and seal the edges by pressing with a fork.

4. **Brush with Egg Wash:**

   - Place the assembled empanadas on a baking sheet lined with parchment paper.

   - Brush the tops of the empanadas with the beaten egg.

5. **Bake:**

- Bake in the preheated oven for 20-25 minutes or until the empanadas are golden brown.

Benefits:

1. **Masa Harina:**

- Adds a nutty flavor and provides dietary fiber, iron, and B vitamins.

2. **Butter:**

- Contributes to the richness and flakiness of the masa dough.

3. **Chicken or Black Beans:**

- Provide protein for muscle health and repair.

4. **Vegetables (Onion, Bell Peppers):**

- Rich in vitamins, minerals, and antioxidants.

- Add flavor and nutrition to the filling.

5. **Ground Cumin, Chili Powder, Smoked Paprika:**

- Spices with potential anti-inflammatory and antioxidant properties.

- Enhance the overall flavor of the filling.

6. **Cilantro:**

   - Adds a fresh and herbaceous flavor.

   - Contains antioxidants and may have antibacterial properties.

7. **Cheese (Monterey Jack or Pepper Jack):**

   - Adds creaminess and a tangy flavor to the filling.

   - Provides calcium and protein.

8. **Egg Wash:**

   - Creates a golden, shiny crust on the empanadas.

Spicy Masa Empanadas offer a flavorful and satisfying combination of masa dough with a spicy, cheesy filling. Enjoy them as a delicious appetizer or a portable snack.

Chocolate Tamales with Raspberry Sauce

Ingredients:

For the Chocolate Masa:

- 2 cups masa harina
- 1 cup unsweetened cocoa powder
- 1 cup granulated sugar
- 1 teaspoon baking powder
- 1/2 teaspoon salt
- 1 cup unsalted butter, softened
- 2 cups warm water or milk

For the Chocolate Filling:

- 1 cup bittersweet chocolate chips or chopped chocolate
- 1/2 cup heavy cream

For the Raspberry Sauce:

- 2 cups fresh or frozen raspberries
- 1/2 cup granulated sugar
- 2 tablespoons water
- 1 tablespoon fresh lime juice

For Wrapping the Tamales:

- Dried corn husks, soaked in warm water until pliable

Method:

1. **Prepare the Chocolate Masa:**

   - In a large bowl, combine masa harina, cocoa powder, granulated sugar, baking powder, and salt.

   - Add softened butter and gradually mix in warm water or milk until a smooth and spreadable consistency is achieved.

2. **Prepare the Chocolate Filling:**

   - In a heatproof bowl, combine bittersweet chocolate and heavy cream.

   - Melt the chocolate over a double boiler or in the microwave, stirring until smooth.

   - Allow the chocolate filling to cool slightly.

3. **Assemble the Chocolate Tamales:**

   - Drain the soaked corn husks and pat them dry.

- Spread a thin layer of the chocolate masa onto the center of each corn husk.

- Spoon a small amount of the chocolate filling onto the masa layer.

- Roll the tamale, enclosing the filling, and fold in the edges to seal.

4. **Steam the Tamales:**

   - Arrange the tamales vertically in a steamer basket, open side up.

   - Steam over boiling water for 1 to 1.5 hours or until the masa is set and easily pulls away from the husk.

5. **Prepare the Raspberry Sauce:**

   - In a saucepan, combine raspberries, granulated sugar, water, and lime juice.

   - Simmer over medium heat until the raspberries break down and the sauce thickens slightly.

   - Remove from heat and strain the sauce to remove seeds, if desired.

6. **Serve:**

- Unwrap the tamales and drizzle them with the raspberry sauce.

- Optionally, garnish with fresh raspberries or a dollop of whipped cream.

Benefits:

1. **Masa Harina:**

- Adds a unique flavor and provides dietary fiber, iron, and B vitamins.

2. **Cocoa Powder:**

- Rich in antioxidants and may have heart-healthy benefits.

- Adds a deep chocolate flavor to the masa.

3. **Butter:**

- Contributes to the richness and moisture of the chocolate masa.

4. **Bittersweet Chocolate:**

- Contains antioxidants and may have mood-boosting properties.

- Adds a rich and velvety texture to the filling.

5. **Heavy Cream:**

   - Adds creaminess and richness to the chocolate filling.

6. **Raspberries:**

   - Packed with vitamins, minerals, and antioxidants.

   - Contribute to the sweet and tart flavor of the sauce.

7. **Granulated Sugar:**

   - Sweetens both the chocolate masa and raspberry sauce.

   - Provides a quick source of energy.

8. **Water or Milk:**

   - Creates a smooth and spreadable consistency in the chocolate masa.

9. **Lime Juice:**

   - Adds acidity to balance the sweetness in the raspberry sauce.

   - Provides vitamin C.

Chocolate Tamales with Raspberry Sauce offer a decadent and fruity twist on traditional tamales, making them a delightful treat for special occasions or dessert.

Masa Pizza with Pico de Gallo

Ingredients:

For the Masa Pizza Dough:

- 2 cups masa harina
- 1 teaspoon baking powder
- 1/2 teaspoon salt
- 1 cup warm water
- 2 tablespoons olive oil

For the Toppings:

- 1 cup tomato sauce or salsa
- 2 cups shredded Mexican cheese blend
- 1 cup cooked and seasoned ground beef or black beans for a vegetarian option
- 1 cup diced bell peppers (mixed colors)
- 1/2 cup diced red onion
- 1 cup sliced cherry tomatoes
- 1 cup sliced black olives
- Fresh cilantro for garnish

Method:

1. **Prepare the Masa Pizza Dough:**

   - In a large bowl, combine masa harina, baking powder, and salt.

   - Gradually add warm water and olive oil, mixing until a soft dough forms.

   - Knead the dough briefly until smooth and pliable.

2. **Roll out the Pizza Dough:**

   - Preheat the oven to 425°F (220°C).

   - Place the masa dough on a parchment paper-lined baking sheet.

   - Roll out the dough into a thin, even layer, creating the pizza crust.

3. **Top the Pizza:**

   - Spread tomato sauce or salsa evenly over the masa pizza crust.

   - Sprinkle shredded Mexican cheese over the sauce.

   - Distribute seasoned ground beef or black beans, diced bell peppers, red onion, cherry tomatoes, and black olives over the cheese.

4. **Bake:**

- Bake in the preheated oven for 15-20 minutes or until the edges are golden and the cheese is melted and bubbly.

5. **Garnish and Serve:**

- Remove the masa pizza from the oven and let it cool for a few minutes.

- Garnish with fresh cilantro before slicing.

Benefits:

1. **Masa Harina:**

- Adds a unique flavor and provides dietary fiber, iron, and B vitamins.

2. **Olive Oil:**

- Contributes to the richness and crispiness of the masa pizza crust.

- Contains healthy monounsaturated fats.

3. **Tomato Sauce or Salsa:**

- Provides a savory base for the pizza.

- Contains lycopene, vitamins, and antioxidants.

4. **Mexican Cheese Blend:**

   - Adds creaminess and a blend of flavors to the pizza.

   - Contains calcium and protein.

5. **Ground Beef or Black Beans:**

   - Provide protein for muscle health and repair.

6. **Bell Peppers, Red Onion, Cherry Tomatoes, Black Olives:**

   - Rich in vitamins, minerals, and antioxidants.

   - Add flavor, color, and nutrition to the pizza.

7. **Fresh Cilantro:**

   - Adds a burst of fresh flavor.

   - Contains antioxidants and may have antibacterial properties.

This Masa Pizza with Pico de Gallo is a fusion of Mexican and Italian flavors, offering a gluten-free crust with vibrant toppings.

Sweet Potato and Black Bean Tamales:

Ingredients:

For the Masa Dough:

- 2 cups masa harina
- 1 teaspoon baking powder
- 1/2 teaspoon salt
- 1/2 cup unsalted butter, softened
- 1 cup vegetable broth
- 1 cup cooked and mashed sweet potatoes

For the Sweet Potato and Black Bean Filling:

- 1 cup black beans, cooked and drained
- 1 cup mashed sweet potatoes
- 1 teaspoon ground cumin
- 1 teaspoon chili powder
- Salt and pepper to taste
- 1/2 cup diced red bell pepper
- 1/4 cup chopped fresh cilantro

For Wrapping the Tamales:

- Dried corn husks, soaked in warm water until pliable

Method:

1. **Prepare the Masa Dough:**

   - In a large bowl, combine masa harina, baking powder, and salt.

   - Add softened butter, vegetable broth, and mashed sweet potatoes.

   - Mix until you have a smooth and spreadable masa dough.

2. **Prepare the Sweet Potato and Black Bean Filling:**

   - In a mixing bowl, combine black beans, mashed sweet potatoes, ground cumin, chili powder, salt, and pepper.

   - Fold in diced red bell pepper and chopped fresh cilantro.

3. **Assemble the Tamales:**

   - Drain the soaked corn husks and pat them dry.

   - Spread a thin layer of the masa dough onto the center of each corn husk.

   - Spoon a portion of the sweet potato and black bean filling onto the masa layer.

- Roll the tamale, enclosing the filling, and fold in the edges to seal.

4. **Steam the Tamales:**

   - Arrange the tamales vertically in a steamer basket, open side up.

   - Steam over boiling water for 1 to 1.5 hours or until the masa is set and easily pulls away from the husk.

5. **Serve:**

   - Unwrap the tamales and serve them hot.

   - Optionally, garnish with additional chopped cilantro and serve with salsa or a drizzle of lime crema.

Benefits:

1. **Masa Harina:**

   - Adds a unique flavor and provides dietary fiber, iron, and B vitamins.

2. **Sweet Potatoes:**

   - Rich in beta-carotene, vitamins, and antioxidants.

   - Provides natural sweetness to the tamales.

3. **Black Beans:**

   - A good source of plant-based protein and fiber.

   - Contains vitamins, minerals, and antioxidants.

4. **Vegetable Broth:**

   - Adds moisture and flavor to the masa dough.

   - May contain nutrients extracted from vegetables during the cooking process.

5. **Red Bell Pepper:**

   - High in vitamin C and antioxidants.

   - Adds a pop of color and a sweet flavor to the filling.

6. **Cumin and Chili Powder:**

   - Spices with potential anti-inflammatory and antioxidant properties.

   - Contribute to the savory and warm flavor profile of the filling.

7. **Cilantro:**

   - Adds a fresh and herbaceous flavor.

- Contains antioxidants and may have antibacterial properties.

These Sweet Potato and Black Bean Tamales offer a flavorful and nutritious twist on traditional tamales, combining the earthy sweetness of sweet potatoes with the protein-rich goodness of black beans. Enjoy these as a delicious and satisfying meal.

Masa-Crusted Fish Tacos

Ingredients:

For the Masa Crust:

- 1 cup masa harina
- 1/2 cup all-purpose flour
- 1 teaspoon baking powder
- 1 teaspoon chili powder
- 1/2 teaspoon cumin
- 1/2 teaspoon garlic powder
- 1/2 teaspoon salt
- 1 cup cold sparkling water
- Vegetable oil for frying

For the Fish:

- 1 pound white fish fillets (such as cod or tilapia), cut into strips
- Salt and pepper to taste
- 1 cup buttermilk
- Lime wedges for serving

For Assembling Tacos:

- Corn or flour tortillas
- Shredded cabbage or lettuce

- Sliced radishes

- Fresh cilantro leaves

- Lime wedges

- Chipotle mayo or your favorite taco sauce

Method:

1. **Prepare the Masa Crust:**

   - In a mixing bowl, whisk together masa harina, all-purpose flour, baking powder, chili powder, cumin, garlic powder, and salt.

   - Gradually add cold sparkling water, whisking until you have a smooth batter.

   - Let the batter rest for 15-20 minutes.

2. **Prepare the Fish:**

   - Season fish fillet strips with salt and pepper.

   - Dip the fish strips into buttermilk to coat, then dredge in the masa batter, ensuring an even coating.

   - In a deep skillet or frying pan, heat vegetable oil over medium-high heat.

- Fry the coated fish strips until golden brown and crispy. Transfer to a paper towel-lined plate to drain excess oil.

3. **Assemble the Tacos:**

   - Warm the tortillas in a dry skillet or microwave.

   - Place a few strips of crispy masa-crusted fish onto each tortilla.

   - Top with shredded cabbage or lettuce, sliced radishes, fresh cilantro leaves, and a drizzle of chipotle mayo or taco sauce.

   - Serve with lime wedges on the side.

Benefits:

1. **Masa Harina:**

   - Adds a unique flavor and provides dietary fiber, iron, and B vitamins.

2. **White Fish (Cod or Tilapia):**

   - A lean source of protein.

   - Contains omega-3 fatty acids and essential nutrients.

3. **Buttermilk:**

   - Adds tanginess and helps tenderize the fish.

   - Contains calcium, vitamin D, and probiotics.

4. **Cabbage or Lettuce:**

   - Low in calories and high in vitamins and fiber.

   - Adds crunch and freshness to the tacos.

5. **Radishes:**

   - Low in calories and a good source of vitamin C.

   - Adds a peppery crunch to the tacos.

6. **Cilantro:**

   - Adds a fresh and herbaceous flavor.

   - Contains antioxidants and may have antibacterial properties.

7. **Lime:**

   - Provides acidity and enhances the overall taste.

   - Rich in vitamin C and adds a citrusy element.

8. **Chipotle Mayo or Taco Sauce:**

- Adds a spicy and savory kick to the tacos.

- Enhances the flavor profile.

Masa-Crusted Fish Tacos offer a delightful combination of crispy texture and bold flavors. Enjoy these tacos as a delicious and satisfying meal that showcases the versatility of masa harina in creating a flavorful crust for the fish.

Masa Gnocchi with Brown Butter Sage Sauce

Ingredients:

For the Masa Gnocchi:

- 2 cups masa harina
- 1 cup ricotta cheese
- 1/2 cup grated Parmesan cheese
- 1 large egg
- 1/2 teaspoon salt

For the Brown Butter Sage Sauce:

- 1/2 cup unsalted butter
- Fresh sage leaves
- Salt and pepper to taste

Optional Garnish:

- Grated Parmesan cheese
- Toasted pine nuts
- Freshly chopped parsley

Method:

1. **Prepare the Masa Gnocchi:**

   - In a large bowl, combine masa harina, ricotta cheese, grated Parmesan cheese, egg, and salt.

   - Mix until a soft dough forms.

   - Divide the dough into smaller portions and roll each portion into a long rope.

   - Cut the ropes into bite-sized pieces to form the gnocchi.

   - Optional: Create ridges on each gnocchi with the back of a fork for texture.

2. **Cook the Masa Gnocchi:**

   - Bring a large pot of salted water to a boil.

   - Drop the gnocchi into the boiling water and cook until they float to the surface (about 2-3 minutes).

   - Remove the gnocchi with a slotted spoon and set aside.

3. **Prepare the Brown Butter Sage Sauce:**

- In a skillet over medium heat, melt the unsalted butter.

- Add fresh sage leaves to the melted butter and let them crisp up.

- Continue cooking until the butter turns golden brown and develops a nutty aroma.

- Season with salt and pepper to taste.

4. **Combine Gnocchi with Sauce:**

- Gently toss the cooked masa gnocchi in the brown butter sage sauce, ensuring they are well coated.

5. **Serve:**

- Plate the masa gnocchi and sage butter sauce.

- Optional: Garnish with grated Parmesan cheese, toasted pine nuts, and freshly chopped parsley.

Benefits:

1. **Masa Harina:**

   - Adds a unique flavor and provides dietary fiber, iron, and B vitamins.

2. **Ricotta Cheese:**

   - Adds creaminess and a mild flavor to the gnocchi.

   - Contains protein and calcium.

3. **Parmesan Cheese:**

   - Provides a savory and nutty flavor.

   - Adds calcium and protein.

4. **Egg:**

   - Contributes to the structure and richness of the gnocchi.

5. **Unsalted Butter:**

   - Enhances the richness and flavor of the brown butter sage sauce.

6. **Sage Leaves:**

   - Add an earthy and savory flavor to the brown butter sauce.

   - May have anti-inflammatory and antioxidant properties.

7. **Salt and Pepper:**

   - Enhance the overall flavor of the dish.

8. **Optional Garnishes:**

   - **Toasted Pine Nuts:** Add a crunchy texture and provide healthy fats.

   - **Freshly Chopped Parsley:** Add freshness and a burst of color.

   - **Grated Parmesan Cheese:** Enhance the cheesy flavor.

Masa Gnocchi with Brown Butter Sage Sauce offers a unique twist on traditional gnocchi, incorporating the rich and nutty flavor of masa harina. Enjoy this dish as a delightful and comforting meal.

Crispy Masa Chicken Tenders

Ingredients:

For the Masa Coating:

- 1 cup masa harina
- 1 cup all-purpose flour
- 1 teaspoon baking powder
- 1 teaspoon garlic powder
- 1 teaspoon onion powder
- 1 teaspoon smoked paprika
- 1/2 teaspoon salt
- 1/4 teaspoon black pepper
- 1 cup cold buttermilk

For the Chicken Tenders:

- 1.5 pounds chicken tenders
- Salt and pepper to taste
- Vegetable oil for frying

For Dipping Sauce:

- 1/2 cup mayonnaise
- 2 tablespoons Dijon mustard
- 1 tablespoon honey

- 1 teaspoon apple cider vinegar

- Salt and pepper to taste

Method:

1. **Prepare the Masa Coating:**

   - In a shallow bowl, combine masa harina, all-purpose flour, baking powder, garlic powder, onion powder, smoked paprika, salt, and black pepper.

   - Pour cold buttermilk into a separate bowl.

2. **Coat the Chicken Tenders:**

   - Season chicken tenders with salt and pepper.

   - Dip each chicken tender into the buttermilk, ensuring it is well coated.

   - Dredge the chicken tender in the masa coating mixture, pressing it to adhere.

3. **Fry the Chicken Tenders:**

   - In a deep skillet or frying pan, heat vegetable oil over medium-high heat.

- Fry the coated chicken tenders in batches until golden brown and crispy.

- Place the cooked tenders on a paper towel-lined plate to absorb excess oil.

4. **Prepare the Dipping Sauce:**

- In a small bowl, whisk together mayonnaise, Dijon mustard, honey, apple cider vinegar, salt, and pepper.

- Adjust the seasoning according to taste.

5. **Serve:**

- Arrange the crispy masa chicken tenders on a serving platter.

- Serve with the dipping sauce on the side.

Benefits:

1. **Masa Harina:**

- Adds a unique flavor and provides dietary fiber, iron, and B vitamins.

2. **All-Purpose Flour:**

   - Contributes to the crispy texture of the coating.

3. **Baking Powder:**

   - Adds lightness and enhances the crispiness of the coating.

4. **Garlic Powder, Onion Powder, Smoked Paprika:**

   - Spices with potential anti-inflammatory and antioxidant properties.

   - Add flavor and depth to the masa coating.

5. **Buttermilk:**

   - Adds tanginess and helps tenderize the chicken.

   - Contains calcium, vitamin D, and probiotics.

6. **Chicken Tenders:**

   - A lean source of protein.

   - Provides essential amino acids and various vitamins and minerals.

7. **Vegetable Oil:**

   - Provides the necessary medium for frying.

   - May contain healthy unsaturated fats.

8. **Dipping Sauce:**

   - **Mayonnaise:** Adds creaminess and richness.

   - **Dijon Mustard:** Adds a tangy and savory kick.

   - **Honey:** Adds sweetness and balances flavors.

   - **Apple Cider Vinegar:** Adds acidity and brightness.

   - **Salt and Pepper:** Enhance the overall flavor.

Crispy Masa Chicken Tenders with a tangy dipping sauce make for a delicious and satisfying snack or meal. Enjoy the crunch of the masa coating paired with the tender and juicy chicken inside.

Chorizo and Potato Pupusas
Ingredients:

For the Pupusa Dough:

- 2 cups masa harina
- 1 1/2 cups warm water
- 1/2 teaspoon salt

For the Chorizo and Potato Filling:

- 1 cup cooked and mashed potatoes
- 1/2 cup cooked chorizo, crumbled
- 1/4 cup diced onion
- 1/4 cup chopped cilantro
- Salt and pepper to taste

For Curtido (Cabbage Slaw):

- 2 cups shredded cabbage
- 1/2 cup shredded carrot
- 1/2 cup thinly sliced red onion
- 1/4 cup chopped fresh cilantro
- 1/2 cup apple cider vinegar
- 1/4 cup water
- 1 teaspoon sugar

- 1 teaspoon salt

For Salsa Roja:

- 2 tomatoes, diced

- 1/2 onion, finely chopped

- 1 jalapeño, seeded and minced

- 2 tablespoons chopped cilantro

- 1 tablespoon lime juice

- Salt and pepper to taste

For Cooking:

- Vegetable oil for greasing the griddle

Method:

1. **Prepare the Pupusa Dough:**
   - In a large bowl, combine masa harina, warm water, and salt.
   - Knead the mixture until you have a soft and pliable dough.
   - Divide the dough into golf ball-sized portions.

2. **Prepare the Chorizo and Potato Filling:**
   - In a mixing bowl, combine mashed potatoes, crumbled chorizo, diced

onion, chopped cilantro, salt, and pepper.

- Mix until the ingredients are well incorporated.

3. **Assemble the Pupusas:**

   - Take a portion of the pupusa dough and flatten it into a disc.

   - Place a spoonful of the chorizo and potato filling in the center.

   - Fold the edges of the dough over the filling, sealing it to form a stuffed pupusa.

4. **Cook the Pupusas:**

   - Preheat a griddle or non-stick skillet over medium-high heat.

   - Grease the surface with vegetable oil.

   - Cook each pupusa for 2-3 minutes on each side or until golden brown and cooked through.

5. **Prepare Curtido (Cabbage Slaw):**

   - In a bowl, combine shredded cabbage, shredded carrot, sliced red onion, chopped cilantro, apple

> cider vinegar, water, sugar, and salt.

- Toss the ingredients together and let the slaw marinate while preparing the other components.

6. **Prepare Salsa Roja:**

- In a separate bowl, combine diced tomatoes, chopped onion, minced jalapeño, chopped cilantro, lime juice, salt, and pepper.

- Mix well to create the salsa.

7. **Serve:**

- Serve the Chorizo and Potato Pupusas warm, accompanied by curtido and salsa roja on the side.

Benefits:

1. **Masa Harina:**

- Adds a unique flavor and provides dietary fiber, iron, and B vitamins.

2. **Potatoes:**

- A good source of complex carbohydrates and dietary fiber.

- Provides essential vitamins and minerals.

3. **Chorizo:**

- Adds a savory and spicy flavor to the filling.

- Contains protein and various spices.

4. **Onion and Cilantro:**

- Add flavor and freshness to the filling and garnishes.

5. **Curtido (Cabbage Slaw):**

- **Cabbage and Carrot:** High in vitamins, minerals, and fiber.

- **Apple Cider Vinegar:** Adds tanginess and may have health benefits.

6. **Salsa Roja:**

- **Tomatoes:** Rich in antioxidants and vitamins.

- **Onion, Jalapeño, Cilantro:** Add flavor and spice.

- **Lime Juice:** Adds acidity and enhances flavors.

7. **Vegetable Oil:**

- Used for greasing the griddle and contributes to the overall texture.

Chorizo and Potato Pupusas with Curtido and Salsa Roja offer a flavorful and satisfying experience, combining the rich taste of chorizo with the comforting texture of masa harina. Enjoy the pupusas with the crunchy curtido and zesty salsa for a delicious meal.

Blue Corn Arepas

Ingredients:

For the Arepa Dough:

- 2 cups blue cornmeal
- 1 cup all-purpose flour
- 1 teaspoon baking powder
- 1 teaspoon salt
- 2 cups warm water
- 2 tablespoons vegetable oil

For the Filling:

- 1 cup shredded cooked chicken
- 1 avocado, sliced
- 1 cup black beans, cooked
- 1 cup crumbled queso fresco or feta cheese
- Fresh cilantro leaves for garnish

For Avocado Crema:

- 1 ripe avocado
- 1/2 cup sour cream or Greek yogurt
- 1 clove garlic, minced
- 2 tablespoons lime juice

- Salt and pepper to taste

Method:

1. **Prepare the Arepa Dough:**

   - In a large bowl, combine blue cornmeal, all-purpose flour, baking powder, and salt.

   - Gradually add warm water and vegetable oil, kneading until you have a soft and smooth dough.

   - Divide the dough into golf ball-sized portions and shape them into thick discs.

2. **Cook the Arepas:**

   - Preheat a skillet or griddle over medium-high heat.

   - Cook each arepa for about 4-5 minutes on each side or until golden brown and cooked through.

   - Allow them to cool slightly before slicing in half horizontally.

3. **Prepare the Filling:**

   - Fill each arepa with shredded cooked chicken, sliced avocado, black beans, and crumbled queso fresco or feta cheese.

- Garnish with fresh cilantro leaves.

4. **Prepare Avocado Crema:**

   - In a blender or food processor, combine ripe avocado, sour cream or Greek yogurt, minced garlic, lime juice, salt, and pepper.

   - Blend until smooth and creamy.

5. **Serve:**

   - Drizzle the assembled arepas with avocado crema.

   - Serve warm and enjoy!

Benefits:

1. **Blue Cornmeal:**

   - Rich in antioxidants, particularly anthocyanins.

   - Provides dietary fiber, vitamins, and minerals.

2. **All-Purpose Flour:**

   - Contributes to the texture and structure of the arepa dough.

3. **Baking Powder:**

   - Adds lightness to the arepa dough.

4. **Warm Water and Vegetable Oil:**

- Create a soft and pliable dough.

5. **Shredded Cooked Chicken:**

- A lean source of protein.

- Provides essential amino acids and nutrients.

6. **Avocado:**

- Rich in healthy monounsaturated fats.

- Provides vitamins, minerals, and antioxidants.

7. **Black Beans:**

- A good source of plant-based protein and fiber.

- Contains vitamins and minerals.

8. **Queso Fresco or Feta Cheese:**

- Adds a salty and creamy element to the filling.

- Provides calcium and protein.

9. **Fresh Cilantro:**

- Adds a burst of fresh flavor.

- Contains antioxidants and may have antibacterial properties.

10. **Avocado Crema:**

   - **Avocado:** Adds creaminess and a rich texture.

   - **Sour Cream or Greek Yogurt:** Adds tanginess and creaminess.

   - **Garlic:** Adds flavor.

   - **Lime Juice:** Adds acidity and brightness.

Blue Corn Arepas with a flavorful and colorful filling, topped with creamy avocado crema, offer a delicious and satisfying meal. Enjoy the unique texture and nutty flavor of blue corn in these versatile and vibrant arepas.

Jalapeño-Cheese Tamales

Ingredients:

For the Masa Dough:

- 2 cups masa harina
- 1 cup vegetable broth
- 1/2 cup unsalted butter, softened
- 1 teaspoon baking powder
- 1/2 teaspoon salt
- 1 cup grated cheddar or Monterey Jack cheese

For the Filling:

- 2 cups cooked and shredded chicken or pork
- 2-3 jalapeños, finely chopped (adjust to taste)
- 1 cup shredded cheddar or Monterey Jack cheese
- 1/4 cup chopped fresh cilantro
- Salt and pepper to taste

For Wrapping the Tamales:

- Dried corn husks, soaked in warm water until pliable

Method:

1. **Prepare the Masa Dough:**

   - In a large bowl, combine masa harina, vegetable broth, softened butter, baking powder, and salt.

   - Mix until you have a soft and spreadable masa dough.

   - Fold in the grated cheddar or Monterey Jack cheese.

2. **Prepare the Filling:**

   - In a separate bowl, mix together shredded chicken or pork, finely chopped jalapeños, shredded cheese, chopped cilantro, salt, and pepper.

3. **Assemble the Tamales:**

   - Drain the soaked corn husks and pat them dry.

   - Spread a thin layer of the masa dough onto the center of each corn husk.

   - Spoon a portion of the filling onto the masa layer.

   - Roll the tamale, enclosing the filling, and fold in the edges to seal.

4. **Steam the Tamales:**

   - Arrange the tamales vertically in a steamer basket, open side up.

   - Steam over boiling water for 1 to 1.5 hours or until the masa is set and easily pulls away from the husk.

5. **Serve:**

   - Unwrap the tamales and serve them warm.

   - Optionally, garnish with additional chopped cilantro and serve with salsa or a drizzle of lime crema.

Benefits:

1. **Masa Harina:**

   - Adds a unique flavor and provides dietary fiber, iron, and B vitamins.

2. **Vegetable Broth:**

   - Adds moisture and flavor to the masa dough.

   - May contain nutrients extracted from vegetables during the cooking process.

3. **Unsalted Butter:**

   - Enhances the richness and flavor of the masa dough.

4. **Baking Powder:**

   - Adds lightness and leavening to the masa dough.

5. **Salt:**

   - Enhances the overall flavor of the masa dough and filling.

6. **Cheddar or Monterey Jack Cheese:**

   - Adds a creamy and cheesy texture to the masa dough and filling.

   - Provides calcium and protein.

7. **Shredded Chicken or Pork:**

   - Adds protein to the filling.

   - Provides essential amino acids and nutrients.

8. **Jalapeños:**

   - Add a spicy kick to the filling.

   - Contain capsaicin, which may have metabolism-boosting properties.

9. **Cilantro:**

- Adds a fresh and herbaceous flavor to the filling.

- Contains antioxidants and may have antibacterial properties.

Jalapeño-Cheese Tamales offer a delightful combination of spicy and cheesy flavors, wrapped in a tender and flavorful masa dough. Enjoy these tamales as a comforting and satisfying meal, perfect for any occasion.

Classic Corn Tortillas:

Ingredients:

- 2 cups masa harina
- 1 1/2 cups warm water
- 1/2 teaspoon salt (optional)

Method:

1. **Prepare the Masa Dough:**
   - In a large bowl, combine masa harina and salt (if using).
   - Gradually add warm water, mixing continuously, until a soft, pliable dough forms.
   - Knead the dough for a few minutes until it becomes smooth.

2. **Divide and Roll:**
   - Divide the masa dough into golf ball-sized portions.
   - Roll each portion into a smooth ball.

3. **Press or Roll Out:**
   - Using a tortilla press or a rolling pin, flatten each ball into a thin, round tortilla.

- Aim for a thickness of about 1/16 to 1/8 inch.

4. **Cook the Tortillas:**

   - Preheat a dry skillet or griddle over medium-high heat.

   - Cook each tortilla for about 30 seconds to 1 minute on each side, or until it develops slight browning and puffiness.

   - Stack the cooked tortillas and keep them warm by covering with a clean kitchen towel.

Benefits:

1. **Masa Harina:**

   - Made from corn that has been soaked in lime water, making it a good source of dietary fiber, iron, and B vitamins.

   - Naturally gluten-free.

2. **Warm Water:**

   - Combines with masa harina to create a pliable dough for forming tortillas.

3. **Salt (Optional):**

   - Adds flavor to the masa dough but can be omitted for a low-sodium version.

4. **Corn Tortillas:**

   - Provide a versatile and staple base for many Mexican dishes.

   - Low in fat and sugar.

   - Gluten-free, making them suitable for individuals with gluten sensitivity or celiac disease.

5. **Tortilla Press or Rolling Pin:**

   - Essential tools for shaping and flattening the masa dough into uniform tortillas.

6. **Dry Skillet or Griddle:**

   - Used for cooking the tortillas, imparting a slightly toasty flavor.

Additional Tips:

- **Consistency of Dough:** The masa dough should be soft, like playdough, and not too sticky. Adjust with more masa harina or water as needed.

- **Uniform Thickness:** Aim for consistent thickness across the tortilla to ensure even cooking.

- **Stacking and Keeping Warm:** Keep the cooked tortillas stacked and covered with a kitchen towel to retain moisture and warmth.

- **Versatility:** Use these classic corn tortillas as the foundation for tacos, enchiladas, quesadillas, or as a side to various Mexican dishes.

Making classic corn tortillas at home allows you to enjoy the authentic flavor and texture of this staple in Mexican cuisine. Customize the size and thickness according to your preferences, and savor the warm, fresh tortillas with your favorite fillings.

Conclusion

As we come to the end of "Modern Methods for Mastering Masa: Discover Revolutionary Techniques, Tempting Recipes, and Thoughtful Reflections on the Timeless Staple," we welcome you to relish the accomplishment of your culinary trip.

Throughout this book, we've been on a mission to discover the mysteries of masa, a beloved and ageless staple with deep origins in cultural traditions.

Our investigation has led us to groundbreaking methodologies, letting you to master the skill of working with masa in ways that defy convention.

We've worked hard to provide you with the knowledge and abilities to enrich your culinary creations, from the fundamentals of making the ideal masa dough to the complexities of generating contemporary masterpieces.

The enticing recipes featured here are more than simply a set of instructions; they are an invitation to savor the rich tapestry of tastes that masa has to offer.

Whether you're making nostalgic classics or experimenting with new variations that push the boundaries of tradition, each recipe celebrates the diversity and adaptability that masa brings to the table.

"Modern Methods for Mastering Masa" is a trip of thought in addition to the gastronomic joys. We've offered tales, anecdotes, and observations about masa's cultural significance, building a stronger connection between the food on your plate and the legacy it symbolizes. As you taste each meal, remember to savor the tales and traditions that go with it.

Finally, we hope you have been inspired by this book to embrace the timeless appeal of masa in your cooking. May the skills you've learned, recipes you've discovered, and thoughts you've pondered bring you joy, creativity, and connection in your culinary pursuits.

"Modern Methods for Mastering Masa" is more than a cookbook; it's an homage to the lasting spirit of a beloved staple, as well as an invitation to transform your kitchen into a space for discovery, invention, and cultural celebration.

Good luck in the kitchen!

www.ingramcontent.com/pod-product-compliance
Lightning Source LLC
Chambersburg PA
CBHW070910260726
48661CB00004B/1678